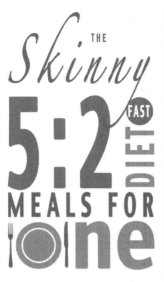

THE
Skinny
5:2 FAST DIET
MEALS FOR
one

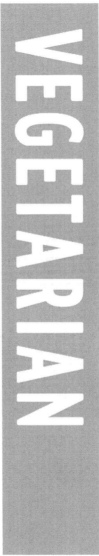
VEGETARIAN

Single serving
fast day recipes
& snacks under
100, 200 & 300
calories

The Skinny 5:2 Fast Diet Vegetarian Meals For One:

Single Serving Fast Day Recipes & Snacks Under 100, 200 & 300 Calories

A Bell & Mackenzie Publication

First published in 2013 by Bell & Mackenzie Publishing

Copyright © Bell & Mackenzie Publishing 2013

ISBN 978-0-9576447-5-5

Disclaimer
The information and advice in this book is intended as a guide only. Any individual should independently seek the advice of a health professional before embarking on a diet. Some recipes may contain nuts or traces of nuts. Those suffering from any allergies associated with nuts should avoid any recipes containing nuts or nut based oils.

Contents

Contents

Contents

The Skinny 5:2 Fast Diet Vegetarian Meals For One

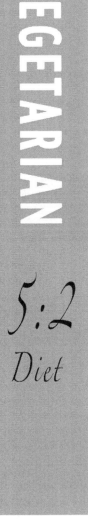

THE
Skinny
5:2 ~FAST~ DIET
MEALS FOR
one

About The *5:2 Diet*

Keep It Simple With Single Servings

So you've made the commitment to start the 5:2 Diet, or maybe you're into your second or third month and looking for some fresh recipe ideas for your fasting days. 'The Skinny 5:2 Fast Diet Vegetarian Meals For One' is packed full of SINGLE SERVING delicious vegetarian recipes under 100, 200 and 300 calories for your fasting days, as well as lots of SINGLE SERVING tasty snack ideas to keep you feeling full and motivated.

There are a multitude of 5:2 recipe books but most cater for multiple servings. This can be extra work adjusting ingredients to single servings – something you shouldn't need to worry about when your efforts are best placed concentrating on your diet. Just plan your fasting days around these SINGLE SERVING recipes and you will be on your way to losing those extra pounds and feeling great.

Each recipe has calorie information so you can keep track of your 500 (women)/600 (men) calorie fasting day limit.

The 5:2 Diet Explained

Imagine a diet where you can eat whatever you want for 5 days a week and only diet for 2. That's what the 5:2 Diet is, and it's revolutionised the way people think about dieting.

By allowing you the freedom to eat normally for MOST of the week and fast by restricting your calorie intake for just TWO non-consecutive days a week (500 calories per day for women/600 for men), you keep yourself motivated and remove that dreaded feeling of constantly denying yourself the food you really want to eat.

It still takes willpower, but it's nowhere near as much of a grind when you know that you have tomorrow to look forward to. It's all about freedom. The ability to be flexible with the days you choose to fast makes the likelihood of you sticking to the diet for a prolonged period, or even indefinitely as a lifestyle choice, much higher than a regime that requires calorie restriction every single day.

Popularised by Dr. Michael J. Mosley, the 5:2 diet plan has been adopted by both health professionals and regular people alike as a way of life, which will change your relationship with dieting and weight loss. What's more, this way of eating is believed to have major health benefits, which could alter your health forever!

How It Works

The concept of fasting is an ancient one and modern science is uncovering evidence that fasting can be an extremely healthy way to shed extra weight. Research has shown that it can reduce levels of IGF-1 (insulin-like growth factor 1, which leads to accelerated ageing), activate DNA repair genes, and reduce blood pressure, cholesterol and glucose levels as well as suggestions of a lower risk of heart disease and cancers.

In short, the 5:2 Diet works by restricting your body to fewer calories than it uses. Most importantly is that it does this in a way that remains healthy and is balanced by eating normally for the other 5 days of the week.

This book has been developed specifically to help you concentrate on the practice of 5:2 through our suggested single serving recipes. However if you want to find out more about the specific details of the science of the subject we would recommend Dr. Michael J. Mosley's work and, as with all diets, you should consider seeking advice from a health professional before starting.

If you are pregnant, breastfeeding, diabetic, suffer from any eating disorder or are under the age of 18 we do not recommend this diet for you. If you suffer from any health issues you should first seek the advice of a health professional before embarking on any form of diet.

What Will This Book Do For Me?

This book will give you a wide choice of delicious, SINGLE SERVING low calorie, easy to prepare meals and snacks that will not only form the basis of your 5:2 Diet plan but will also open your eyes to a new lifestyle choice.

The 5:2 Diet if followed correctly, will help you lose weight and in the long term, improve your overall health and immune system.

This book has been designed to help you through your 5:2 Diet journey by providing a wide selection of easy to prepare recipes and snack ideas FOR ONE to keep you motivated and your engine stoked during your fasting days. What makes the 5:2 Diet so good is that it's only a part time diet. Because you can eat what you want for the other 5 days a week, you'll be much more likely to stick with it over time and enjoy the long term health and weight benefits.

When Can I Expect To See Results?

By the end of your first week in most cases! Obviously everybody is different, but where someone is carrying extra weight they will normally see a reduction in the first week of embarking on the 5:2 Diet. Typically many will see a greater weight loss at the beginning, followed by a slowing down then eventually settling around a stable healthy weight.

Taking It Week By Week

The 5:2 Diet can work for you whatever your lifestyle. Each week you should think carefully about which days are likely to be best suited to your fasting days and then stick with it. You can change your days each week or keep in a regular routine, whichever suits you best. Ideally your fasting days should be non-consecutive. This gives you the opportunity to stay motivated by eating normally the following day, although it can be acceptable to fast for 2 days consecutively if you are feeling particularly inspired.

Of course, reducing your calorie intake for two days will take some getting used to and inevitably there will be hunger pangs to start with, but you'll be amazed at how quickly your body adapts to your new style of eating and, far from gorging the day after your fasting day, you'll find you simply enjoy the luxury of eating normally.

Whether you live on your own or part of a family, the single serving recipes will make it easy for you to stick to your fasting days.

How Will I Manage My Calorie Intake?

There are a number of different approaches to managing your 500 calorie intake (600 for men) on your fast days depending on your personal preferences and lifestyle.

OPTION 1: Skip breakfast, eat lunch & dinner.

OPTION 2: Skip lunch, eat breakfast and dinner.

OPTION 3: Eat little and often throughout the day.

There is much research and debate about the health benefits and risks of skipping meals, however the beauty of the 5:2 Diet is that the fasting occurs only for 2 days of the week with the remaining 5 reserved for 'normal' eating and recommended daily calorie intakes (1900-2000 for women, 2400-2500 for men). The point being that there is not a prolonged period of starving the body of calories, and eating balanced meals like those included in this book ensures that nutrition is still provided on the fasting days.

Portion Sizes

The size of the portion that you put on your plate will significantly affect your weight loss efforts. Filling your plate with over-sized portions will obviously increase your calorie intake and hamper your dieting efforts.

It's important that with all meals, both on your fasting and normal eating days, you use a correct sized portion, which generally is the size of your clenched fist.

You will be surprised at how quickly you will adopt this as the 'norm' as the weeks go by and you will begin to stop over-eating.

Measurements

All recipes are for one serving but can easily be increased if you are cooking for others too. As with portion sizes, stick with the recommended measurements of ingredients. Altering these will affect your calorie intake and therefore your ultimate weight loss.

Choosing Your Fast Days

Give yourself the best possible chance of success by choosing your fast days in advance and sticking to them. As we have already said, we recommend choosing two non-consecutive fasting days so that you only have one 24-hour period at a time where you have to concentrate on limiting your calories.

It makes sense to choose your fast days sensibly based on your own particular lifestyle. For example, for many, a Friday night may involve takeaway food after a hard week at work. If this is your ritual, then avoid this as your fasting day. Similarly if you meet up with friends during the week or have a business event that is likely to involve lunch or dinner then choose an alternative day. You can alter the days each week but just remember to check your calendars and prepare in advance.

Eat, Chew, Wait

In today's fast moving society many of use have adopted an unhealthy habit of eating. We eat as quickly as possibly without properly giving our bodies the chance to digest and feel full. Not only is this bad for your digestive system, but our bodies begin to relate food to just fuel instead of actually enjoying what we are eating.

Some simple tips for eating which may help you on your fasting days:

Eat. Take it slow. There is no rush.

Chew. It sounds obvious but you should properly chew your food and swallow only when it's broken down and you have enjoyed what you have tasted.

Wait. Before reaching for second helpings wait 5-10 minutes and let your body tell you whether you are still hungry. More often than not, the answer will be no and you will be satisfied with the meal you have had. A glass of water before each meal will help you with any cravings for more.

Nutrition

All of the recipes in this collection are balanced low calorie meals and snacks for one, which should keep you feeling full on your fasting days.

In any diet, it is important to balance your food between proteins, good carbs, dairy, fruit and vegetables.

Protein. Keeps you feeling full and is also essential for building body tissue. Vegetarian protein can be found in wholegrain, nuts, seeds, eggs, beans and pulses.

Carbohydrates. Not all carbs are good and generally they are high in calories, which makes them difficult to include in a calorie limiting diet. Carbs are a good source of energy for your body as they are converted more easily into glucose (sugar) providing energy. Try to eat 'good carbs' which are high in fibre and nutrients e.g. whole fruits and veg, nuts, seeds, whole grain cereals, beans and legumes.

Dairy. Dairy products provide you with vitamins and minerals. Cheeses can be very high in calories and some contain animal rennet, but other products such as low fat

Greek yoghurt, crème fraiche and skimmed milk are all good.

Fruit & Vegetables. Eat your five a day. There is never a better time to fill your 5 a day quota. Not only are fruit and veg very healthy, they also fill up your plate and are ideal snacks when you are feeling hungry.

Some 5:2 Tips

Avoid too much exercise on your fasting days. Eating less is likely to make you feel a little weaker, certainly to start with, so don't put the pressure on yourself to exercise.

Avoid alcohol on your fasting days. Not only is alcohol packed with calories, it could also have a greater effect on you than usual as you haven't eaten as much.

Don't give up! Even if you find your fasting days tough to start with, stick with it. Remember you can eat what you like tomorrow without having to feel guilty.

Drink plenty of water throughout the day. Water is the best friend you have on your fasting days. It's good for you, has zero calories, and will fill you up and help stop you feeling hungry.

When you are eating each meal, put your fork down between bites – it will make you eat more slowly and you'll feel fuller on less food.

Drink a glass of water before and also with your meal. Again this will help you feel fuller.

Brush your teeth immediately after your meal to discourage yourself from eating more.

Have clear motivations. Think about what you are trying to achieve and stick with it. Remember you can eat what you want tomorrow.

If unwanted food cravings do strike, acknowledge them, then distract yourself. Go out for a walk, phone a friend, play with the kids, or paint your nails.

Whenever hunger hits, try waiting 15 minutes and ride out the cravings. You'll find they pass and you can move on with your day.

Remember - feeling hungry is not a bad thing. We are all so used to acting on the smallest hunger pangs that we forget what it's like to feel genuinely hungry. Feeling hungry for a couple of days a week is not going to harm you. Learn to 'own' your hunger and take control of how you deal with it.

If you feel you can't do it by yourself then get some support. Encourage a friend or partner to join you on the 5:2 Diet. Having someone to talk things through with can be a real help.

Get moving. Being active isn't a necessity for the 5:2 Diet to have results but as with all diets increased activity will complement your weight loss efforts. Think about what you are doing each day: choose the stairs instead of the lift, walk to the shops instead of driving. Making small changes will not only help you burn calories but will make you feel healthier and more in control of your weight loss.

Don't beat yourself up! If you have a bad day forget about it, don't feel guilty. Recognise where you went wrong and move on. Tomorrow is a new day and you can start all over again. Fast for just two days a week and you'll see results. Guaranteed!

Calorie Conscious Side Suggestions

If you want to make any of the recipes or snacks in this book more substantial you may want to add an accompaniment to them. Here's a list of some key side vegetables, salad, noodles etc which you may find useful when working out your calories.

All calories are per 100g/3 ½ oz. Rice and noodle measurements are cooked weights

Asparagus: 20   cals

Beansprouts: 30 cals

Brussel Sprouts: 42 cals

Butternut Squash: 45 cals

Cabbage: 30 cals

Carrots: 41 cals

Cauliflower: 25 cals

Celery: 14 cals

Courgette/zucchini: 16 cals

Cucumber: 15   cals

Egg noodles: 62 cals

Green beans: 81 cals

Leeks: 61 cals

Long grain rice: 140 cals

Mixed salad leaves: 17 cals

Mixed salad leaves: 30 cals

Mushrooms: 22 cals

Pak choi; 13 cals

Parsnips: 67 cals

Peas: 64 cals

Pepper (bell): 20 cals

Potatoes: 75 cals

Rocket: 17 cals

Shirataki 'Miracle' noodles: 30 cals

Spinach: 23 cals

Sweet Potato: 86 cals

Sweet corn: 86 cals

Tomatoes: 18 cals

THE Skinny

5:2 FAST DIET

MEALS FOR one

VEGETARIAN

Light Bite Recipes Under 100 Calories

Mushroom Egg White Omelette

Serves: 1 Calories: 88

Ingredients:

3 egg whites

50g/2oz mushrooms

Salt & pepper to taste

1 tbsp chopped flat leaf parsley

1 slice (about 10g) low fat vegetarian cheddar cheese, chopped

Method:

Gently sauté the mushrooms in small a frying pan with a little low cal cooking spray for a few minutes. Break and separate the egg whites into a bowl, season well and then tip the softened mushrooms, parsley and cheese into the egg whites. Add a little more low cal spray to the frying pan and pour in the egg and mushroom mixture. Cook until golden brown on the underside. Flip the omelette, cook for a minute or two more and serve.

Cucumber Cakes

Serves: 1 Calories: 97

Ingredients:

½ cucumber

1 tbsp low fat crème fraiche

1 tbsp low fat houmous

1 tbsp chopped dill

Method:

Cut the cucumber into 4 thick slices. Mix the crème fraiche and houmous together and spread equally over the top of each cucumber slice. Sprinkle the dill over the top and serve.

Thai Carrot Noodles

Serves: 1 Calories: 91

Ingredients:

1 tbsp lime juice

½ tsp brown sugar

1 shallot, finely chopped

½ red chilli, deseeded and finely chopped

1 carrot, cut into fine matchsticks

1 tbsp freshly chopped mint

50g/2oz Shirataki 'miracle' noodles

Method:

Cook the noodles as per the manufacturers instructions. Mix together the lime juice, sugar, shallots, chillies and carrots. Add to the noodles and sprinkle with chopped mint.

Balsamic Aubergine & Rocket Salad

Serves: 1 Calories: 96

Ingredients:

½ aubergine/egg plant, cut into small chunks

1 tbsp balsamic vinegar

50g/2oz rocket

Salt & pepper to taste

Low cal cooking spray

Method:

Pre-heat oven to 200C/180C fan/gas 6. Spray the aubergine with low cal cooking oil. Season and spoon over the balsamic vinegar. Place on a baking tray and roast for 20-30 mins until soft and browned. Mix with the rocket and serve.

Lime Courgette Snack

Serves: 1 Calories: 94

Ingredients:

1 courgette/zucchini, sliced

½ red chilli, deseeded and finely chopped

50g/2oz spinach

1 tbsp lime juice

Low cal cooking oil

Method:

Heat a little low cal cooking spray in a frying pan and cook the courgette slices. Season well, add the chilli, spinach and lemon juice; cook for a minute longer until the spinach wilts and serve.

Cauliflower & Capers

Serves: 1 Calories: 95

Ingredients:

¼ head large cauliflower

½ carrot, grated

½ red onion, finely chopped

1 tsp capers, chopped

1 tbsp chopped parsley

2 tsp white wine vinegar

½ tsp Dijon mustard

1 tbsp low fat mayonnaise

1 tbsp warm water

Method:

Split the cauliflower into little florets so that none are bigger than 2cm/1inch. Add to the carrots, red onion, capers and chopped parsley. Mix together the white wine vinegar, water, Dijon mustard and mayonnaise. Season well and toss through the cauliflower salad.

Rosemary Olives

Serves: 1 Calories: 92

Ingredients:

50g/2oz green olives

½ tsp chopped fresh rosemary

1 sundried tomato, finely chopped

½ tsp olive oil

Pinch of crushed sea salt

1 garlic clove, finely chopped

Method:

Toss all the ingredients together and chill.

Chilli Asparagus Spears

Serves: 1 Calories: 98

Ingredients:

10 Asparagus spears

½ red chilli finely chopped

Low cal cooking spray

1 tsp balsamic vinegar

Method:

Trim the thick woody end from the asparagus spears. Cook the asparagus in salted boiling water for 2-3 minutes. Drain and then rinse in cold water. Dry and set to one side. Cover the spears with a little low cal cooking spray and place in a hot fry frying pan. Cook for 3 minutes to brown the spears, season and then add the chilli and balsamic vinegar to the pan for a minute longer. Mix well and serve.

Melon Fruit Cup

Serves: 1 Calories: 89

Ingredients:

¼ melon flesh, cubed

2 tbsp orange juice

Pinch brown sugar

40g/1 ½ oz raspberries

Method:

Gently combine all the ingredients together and serve in a cup.

Minted Grapefruit

Serves: 1 Calories: 95

Ingredients:

1 pink grapefruit

2 shallots, finely sliced

Pinch soft brown sugar

1 tbsp freshly chopped mint

1 tbsp freshly chopped coriander/cilantro

Low cal cooking spray

Method:

Peel and cut the grapefruit into slices. Gently sauté the chopped shallots in a little low cal cooking spray for a minute or two with a pinch of sugar. Arrange the grapefruit slices on a plate and scatter over the shallots and chopped herbs.

Cauliflower Cheese

Serves: 1 Calories: 94

Ingredients:

100g/3 ½ oz cauliflower florets

25g/1oz grated low fat vegetarian cheddar cheese

Pinch of nutmeg

Salt & pepper to taste

Method:

Preheat oven to 375°F/190°C/gas mark 5

Break the cauliflower head into small florets and wash under a cold tap. Place in a small ovenproof dish, season and grate the cheese over the top. Add a pinch of nutmeg and bake for 20-30 mins until brown on top.

Spicy Watermelon Salad

Serves: 1 Calories: 60

Ingredients:

1 slice watermelon

1 small red chilli, deseeded and finely chopped

1 tsp freshly chopped coriander/cilantro

1 tbsp red onion, finely chopped

1 tsp lime juice

Method:

Cube the watermelon and combine with chilli, coriander/cilantro and lime juice for a sweet crunchy snack with a kick.

White Bean Salad

Serves: 1 Calories: 99

Ingredients:

75g/3oz tinned cannellini beans

1 tbsp spring onions/scallions chopped

1 medium tomato, chopped

1 tsp lemon juice

Salt & pepper to taste

1 tbsp fresh chopped flat leaf parsley

Method:

Drain the beans and combine in a bowl with the spring onions, parsley, tomato and lemon juice. Season well and serve.

Raw Asparagus & Mushroom Salad

Serves: 1 Calories: 99

Ingredients:

6 asparagus spears

40g/1½ oz mushrooms, sliced

1 tsp fresh chopped flat leaf parsley

1 tsp lemon juice

½ tsp vegetarian parmesan-style grated cheese

½ tsp olive oil

Salt & pepper to taste

Method:

Wash and remove any tough stalks from the asparagus and discard. Thinly slice the tender stalks. Wash the mushrooms and again thinly slice. Season and combine all ingredients in a bowl topped with grated parmesan.

Boozy Strawberries

Serves: 1 Calories: 83

Ingredients:

¼ cantaloupe melon flesh

2 tbsp rose wine

1 tsp rose water

50g/2oz strawberries, sliced

Method:

Cut the melon into strips and place in a bowl with the strawberries, rose water and wine. Combine well and arrange neatly on a plate.

Iced Tomato & Lettuce Snack

Serves: 1 Calories: 81

Ingredients:

100g/3 ½ oz vine ripened tomatoes

1 tsp tomato puree/paste

1 spring onion/scallion

1 stick celery

1/2 clove garlic, crushed

1 tsp fresh chopped flat leaf parsley

½ baby gem lettuce, shredded

Method:

In a food processor pulse together the tomatoes, celery, spring onions and tomato paste. Place in the freezer and leave for 30-40 minutes. Place the iced mixture back into the food processor and pulse briefly to make into an icy slush. Place the shredded lettuce in a bowl and arrange the slush on top. Season, sprinkle with parsley and serve.

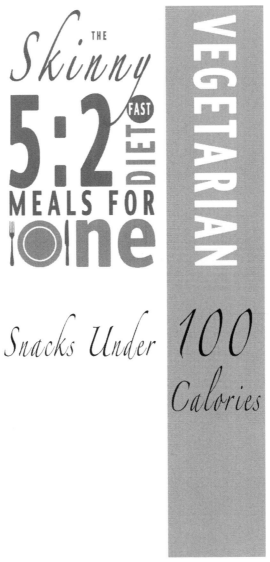

Here's a list of useful 'grab & go' snack ideas to keep you on track when you're feeling hungry on your fast days and need an instant boost.

Chocolate Banana: 100 calories

Half a frozen banana dipped in 2 squares of melted dark chocolate.

Frozen Grapes: 86 calories

125g/4oz of green or black grapes frozen.

Blueberry Yoghurt: 91 calories

100g/3 ½ oz blueberries mixed with 2 tbsp of fat free Greek yoghurt.

Chocolate Strawberries: 72 calories

5 medium strawberries dipped in 2 squares of melted dark chocolate.

Spiced Apple: 95 calories

1 medium apple, cored & sliced; sprinkled with ½ tsp brown sugar and 1 tsp cinnamon. Bake in the oven until soft.

Latte: 93 calories

250ml/1 cup skimmed milk with 1 shot of espresso coffee.

Houmous & Veg Dips: 71 calories

2 tbsp low fat houmous with 1 carrot & 1 stalk celery cut into crudités.

Pistachios: 85 calories

1 small cup (around 25 nuts).

Sweet Potato Fries: 95 calories

1 small sweet potato, peeled and sliced into thin matchsticks tossed in a little low cal cooking spray and cooked in the oven at

375F/190C/gas mark 5 for 10 mins turning twice.

Olives: 50 calories

6 Kalamata olives.

Asparagus & Boiled Egg: 98 calories

1 free range egg cooked to perfection (place egg in a pan of cold water, bring to the boil and simmer for exactly 3 minutes).

2 asparagus tips for dipping - steam the asparagus for 3-5 minutes.

Carrot & Raisin Salad: 100 calories

1 cup of shaved carrot mixed with 25g/1oz raisins and a splash of balsamic vinegar.

Baked Beans In Tomato Sauce: 70 calories

Choose the low salg and sugar canned options and measure 100g.

Asian Broccoli: 50 calories

50g/2oz broccoli. Cut the broccoli into florets. Heat a little low cal spray in a wok or large frying pan and toss in the broccoli, 1 thumb sized piece of fresh ginger (finely chopped) and 1 tbsp of soy sauce. Cook on a high heat for 5 mins stirring frequently.

Grapefruit: 45 calories

1/2 large pink grapefruit with 1 tsp sugar.

Popcorn: 97 calories

2 cups of air popped corn. Add 1 tsp of sugar.

Popcorn Cheese: 94 calories

2 cups of air popped corn. Add 1 tsp of grated parmesan cheese and a pinch of salt.

Grilled Sweet Peppers: 82 calories

1/2 each of green, red and yellow sweet peppers. Slice into 1 inch strip, mix in a bowl with 1 tbsp balsamic vinegar and place under a medium grill until tender.

Wasabi Peas: 68 calories

3 tbsp wasabi peas.

Pumpkin Seeds: 100 calories

2 tbsps of pumpkin seeds

Edamame Beans: 100 calories

1/4 cup of steamed edamame beans (4 mins) with a pinch of crushed sea salt.

Hardboiled egg: 78 calories

Place 1 medium free range egg in a pan of cold water and bring to the boil. Continue to simmer for 5 mins then allow to cool.

Frozen Banana: 90 calories

Peel and place in the freezer for 2 hours.

Pickled Gherkins: 50 calories

300g/12oz pickled gherkins.

Toast & Marmite: 100 calories

1 slice of wholemeal toast, low fat spread and marmite spread thinly.

Portabella Mushroom & Feta: 100 calories

1 medium portabella mushroom cap with 1 tsp low fat vegetarian feta-style cheese. Fill the mushroom cap with feta, season and gently grill for 10 mins.

Cottage Cheese & Celery: 75 calories

75g/3oz low fat natural cottage cheese with 3 celery sticks.

Guacamole & Chips: 96 calories

1 tbsp of low fat guacamole with 8 tortilla chips.

Crackers & Peanut Butter: 93 calories

2 crackers/crackerbread thinly spread with peanut butter.

Strawberries & Goat's Cheese: 98 calories

10 strawberries dipped in 2 tsp low fat vegetarian goat's cheese.

Cherries & Fromage Frais: 97 calories

60ml/ ¼ cup low fat fromage frais + 5 cherries.

Cinnamon Orange: 80 calories

1 medium orange, peeled and split into segments. In a bowl mix together 1 tsp of lemon juice, 1 tsp orange juice and a pinch of cinnamon. Pour over orange segments and serve.

Paprika Eggs: 100 calories

I medium hard boiled egg, sliced. Cover the egg in 1 tsp olive oil and spindle with paprika.

Cottage Cheese Salad: 95 calories

50g/2oz low-fat natural cottage cheese topped with 3 chopped spring onions/scallions. Chop ½ red pepper, mix and serve.

Tricolore: 94 calories

1 slice of low fat mozzarella cheese, 3 cherry tomatoes and 3 fresh basil leaves, Salt & pepper to serve.

Cottage Cheese & Pineapple: 72 calories

50g low fat cottage cheese with 50g fresh pineapple.

Black-eyed Beans: 90 calories

50g/2oz tinned beans, 1 medium chopped tomato, 1 tbsp chopped onion and 1/2 tsp minced garlic, combine. Season and serve.

Warm Goats Cheese with Sugar Snap Peas

100g/3 ½ oz sugar snap peas steamed for 4 minutes. Warm 20g/ ¾ oz vegetarian goat's cheese for 10 secs in a microwave.

Celery & Cream Cheese; 68 calories

3 celery stalks with 2 tsp low-fat cream cheese.

Honey Yoghurt: 79 calories

120ml/ ½ cup fat free Greek yoghurt with 1 tsp runny honey.

Cheesy tomatoes: 89 calories

2 plum tomatoes split in half, topped with 1 tbsp breadcrumbs and 1 tbsp vegetarian parmesan-style cheese. Bake in a hot oven for 45-60 mins.

Apple Cider Cucumber salad: 42 calories

100g/3 ½ oz diced cucumber mixed with 2 tbsp chopped red onion and 1 tbsp cider vinegar.

Chickpea, Lemon & Spring Onions: 78 calories

50g/2oz tinned chickpeas, 1 tbsp lemon juice, 3 chopped spring onions/scallions. Combine all ingredients and serve.

Curried Sweet Potato: 90 calories

100g/3 ½ oz diced sweet potato, 1 tsp curry powder. Cook the sweet potato for 6 mins in a microwave then mash with curry powder and salt & pepper to taste.

THE

Skinny

5:2 FAST DIET

MEALS FOR one

VEGETARIAN

Recipes Under 200 Calories

Vegetable Chilli Snack Bowl

Serves: 1 Calories: 170

Ingredients:

1 garlic clove, crushed

1 red chilli, deseeded and finely chopped

½ tsp each ground cumin & coriander/cilantro

75g/3oz fresh mushrooms, sliced

100g/3 ½oz each chopped tomatoes & kidney beans

70g/3oz green beans, chopped

1 tbsp low fat crème fraiche

1 tsp chopped chives

Salt & pepper to taste

Low cal cooking spray

Method:

Gently sauté the garlic and chilli in a little low cal spray for 2-3 mins. Add the cumin, coriander, mushrooms, tomatoes, kidney beans, green beans and 2 tbsp water. Stir well, season and leave to simmer for 10-15 minutes or until all the veg is tender and the chilli is nice and thick. If you prefer more of a crunch add the green beans later in the cooking. Dollop the crème fraiche into the middle of the chilli and serve with the chives sprinkled over the top.

Roasted Japanese Aubergine

Serves: 1 Calories: 194

Ingredients:

1 aubergine/egg plant

½ tsp golden caster sugar

1 tsp lemon juice

2 spring onions/scallions, cut into fine lengths

1 tbsp each miso paste & sake

50g/2oz rocket

Salt & pepper to taste

1 lime wedge

Low cal cooking spray

Method:

Pre-heat the oven to 200C/fan 180C/gas 6.

Cut the aubergine/eggplant in half lengthways. Brush the exposed flesh with a little low cal cooking spray and season well. Place on a baking tray and cook for 15-20 minutes until the flesh is tender.

Heat the grill up and mix together the sake, miso, sugar and lemon juice and brush it all onto the roasted aubergine flesh. Place under the hot grill and cook for 2 minutes or until the flesh turns golden. Serve with the rocket, spring onions and a wedge of lime.

Super Simple Squash Curry Snack

Serves: 1 Calories: 179

Ingredients:

½ onion, sliced

2 tsp curry paste

125g/4oz butternut squash, peeled and cubed

1 tomato, quartered

50g/2oz spinach, chopped

120ml/ ½ cup water

1 tsp chopped coriander/cilantro

Salt & pepper to taste

Low cal cooking spray

Method:

Gently sauté the onion in a little low cal spray for a few minutes. Add the curry paste and cook for a further minute before adding the squash, tomatoes and water. Season, stir well, cover and leave to simmer for 10 minutes or until the squash is tender. Add the spinach and warm through for a minute. Serve with the chopped coriander sprinkled over the top.

Tomato & Basil Spaghetti

Serves: 1 Calories: 191

Ingredients:

50g/2oz spaghetti

1 garlic clove, crushed

100g/3 ½ oz tinned chopped tomatoes

½ vegetable stock cube

1 tsp tomato purée/paste

½ tsp sugar

1 tsp dried basil

1 tsp fresh chopped basil

Low cal cooking spray

Method:

Cook the spaghetti in boiling salted water until tender. Meanwhile gently sauté the garlic in a little low cal cooking spray for 1 minute. Crumble the stock cube and add it to the garlic along with the chopped tomatoes, tomato puree, sugar and dried basil; simmer for a few minutes. When the spaghetti is cooked, drain and place into the tomato pan. Combine well. Sprinkle with the fresh basil and serve.

Fried Zucchini & Egg

Serves: 1 Calories: 197

Ingredients:

200g/7oz courgettes/zucchini, chopped

100g/3 ½ oz cherry tomatoes

1 garlic clove, crushed

1 free range egg

1 tbsp chopped fresh basil

Salt & pepper to taste

Low cal cooking spray

Method:

Cut the tomatoes into halves and gently sauté along with the courgettes and garlic in a little low cal spray for 5 minutes. Break the egg into the pan, season, cover and leave to cook for 2 minutes or until the egg is cooked as you like it. Serve with the fresh basil sprinkled over.

Lemon Spaghetti

Serves: 1 Calories: 157

Ingredients:

50g/2oz celeriac, peeled

1 carrot, peeled

½ leek

1 red pepper/bell pepper

½ garlic clove

1 celery stick, chopped

75g/3oz spaghetti

½ tsp celery seeds

1 tbsp each low fat crème fraiche and lemon juice

Low cal cooking oil

Salt & pepper to taste

Method:

Cut the celeriac, carrots and pepper into thin matchsticks and sauté in a little low cal spray for 2-3 minutes. Cook the spaghetti in salted boiling water until tender. Mix the vegetables and spaghetti together and stir the crème fraiche and lemon juice through. Heat gently for a minute or two. Season and serve with chopped celery over the top.

Peanut Noodles

Serves: 1 Calories: 196

Ingredients:

75g/3oz fine egg noodles

1 tsp sesame oil

2 tsp crunchy peanut butter

1 tbsp soy sauce

1 tsp white wine vinegar

50g/2oz cucumber, grated

Pinch caster sugar

2 spring onions/scallions, cut into lengthways strips

1 carrot, peeled and grated

Salt & pepper to taste

Method:

Cook the noodles in salted boiling water until tender. Meanwhile mix together the sesame oil, peanut butter, soy sauce, honey and sugar. Combine the peanut sauce with the noodles, spring onions, carrot and grated cucumber. Season and serve with the sliced spring onions sprinkled over the top.

Breakfast Muffin

Serves: 1 Calories: 193

Ingredients:

½ wholemeal muffin

1 free range egg

1 portabella mushroom, sliced

½ beef steak/heirloom tomato, sliced

½ cup vegetable stock

Low fat spread

Salt & pepper to taste

Method:

Place the stock in a frying pan and gently poach the egg and mushrooms in the stock for a few minutes until the egg is cooked to your liking. Meanwhile toast the muffin and tomato under a grill, the muffin will be ready first. 'Butter' with a scrape of low fat spread and set to one side. When everything is cooked load up the muffin with the egg, mushrooms, tomatoes and chopped chives. Season and serve.

Stuffed Mushrooms

Serves: 1 Calories: 188

Ingredients:

2 portabella mushrooms

2 spring onions/scallions

1 slice low cal bread

50g/2oz low fat vegetarian cheddar, grated

½ tsp dried basil

½ clove garlic

Salt & pepper to taste

Low cal cooking oil

Method:

Whizz the bread, garlic, spring onions and basil in a food processor to make herb breadcrumbs. Season the mushrooms and spray with a little low cal oil. Place under a preheated grill and cook for a few minutes until tender. In the meantime combine the breadcrumb mixture and cheese. Divide equally on top of the two mushrooms, Season and place back under the grill for a few minutes until the cheese melts.

Lime Grapefruit & Coconut Salad

Serves: 1 Calories: 191

Ingredients:

25g/1oz grated coconut

½ clove garlic, crushed

½ red onion, sliced

½ grapefruit

1 handful cress or alfalfa sprouts

1 tsp soy sauce

1 tbsp lime juice

1 tbsp water

Salt & pepper to taste

Method:

Gently brown the grated coconut in a dry frying pan for 2-3 minutes and remove from the pan. Coat the pan with a little low cal spray and gently sauté the onion and garlic for a few minutes until soft. Add to the grated coconut. Peel and segment the grapefruit and arrange on a plate. Sprinkle the cress over the top and add the coconut mixture. Season and serve.

No Nicoise Pasta Salad

Serves: 1 Calories: 177

Ingredients:

50g/2oz each penne pasta & chopped green beans

100g/3 ½ oz cherry tomatoes, halved

50g/2oz black pitted olives, sliced

1 tbsp fresh chopped basil leaves

1 tsp each olive oil & lemon juice

½ clove garlic, crushed

4 radishes, sliced

1 free range egg, quartered

½ baby gem lettuce, shredded

Salt & pepper to taste

Low cal cooking oil

Method:

Cook the penne in salted boiling water until tender and hard boil the egg in boiling water. Leave to cool, peel and quarter. Gently sauté the green beans in a little low cal cooking spray. Mix the olive oil, garlic and lemon juice together and toss with the shredded lettuce, radishes, olives and tomatoes. Arrange all the ingredients on a plate, season and sprinkle with fresh basil.

Bombay Potatoes

Serves: 1 Calories: 150

Ingredients:

1 tsp sunflower oil

¼ tsp mustard seeds

½ tsp mild chilli powder

½ tsp turmeric powder

100g/3 ½ oz potatoes, boiled and cubed

½ tsp salt

1 tbsp fresh chopped coriander/cilantro

Method:

Mix the chilli and turmeric in a cup with a little water to form a paste.

Heat the oil in a pan. When it is hot add the mustard seeds and cook for a minute or two until they start to pop. Add the spice paste to the mustard seeds along with the boiled cubed potatoes and cook for a few minutes until the potatoes are completely covered in the spice mix and piping hot. Sprinkle with coriander to serve.

Saag Aloo

Serves: 1 Calories: 197

Ingredients:

60ml/ ¼ cup low-fat coconut milk

½ onion, chopped

250g/9oz spinach leaves

½ green chilli chopped

75g/3oz potatoes, cubed

100g/3½oz tinned chopped tomatoes

1 tsp mild curry powder

½ tsp garam masala

¼ tsp each salt & sugar

Low cal cooking spray

Method:

Gently saute the onion and green chilli in a little low cal spray for a few minutes. Add the potatoes and curry powder, fry for a minute longer then add the tomatoes, spinach, salt & pepper. Cover and leave to simmer gently until the potatoes are tender. Remove from heat, stir through the coconut milk and serve.

Cooked Breakfast

Serves: 1 Calories: 177

Ingredients:

1 large field mushroom

2 tomatoes, halved

1 tsp dried oregano or basil

1 garlic clove, crushed

75g/3oz spinach

1 free range egg

Low cal cooking spray

Salt & pepper to taste

Method:

Pre-heat oven to 200C/180C fan/gas 6.

Place the mushroom and halved tomatoes in a small oven-proof dish. Season and cover with a little low cal spray. Spread the garlic and oregano over the mushroom and tomatoes then bake for 8-10 mins. While this is cooking put the spinach in a colander and quickly pour some boiling water through it over a sink. Add the wilted spinach to the mushroom dish leaving a little 'well' to crack the egg in to. Cook in the oven for a further 8-10 mins or until the tomatoes are tender and the egg is cooked as you like it.

Shredded Cabbage & Coconut Cream

Serves: 1 Calories: 198

Ingredients:

100g/3 ½oz small salad potatoes

½ tsp mustard seeds

½ tsp cumin seeds

½ tsp dried chilli flakes

½ onion, chopped

½ pointed cabbage, shredded

1 tbsp lemon juice

2 tsp low fat coconut cream

1 tbsp chopped fresh coriander/cilantro

Low cal cooking spray

Salt & pepper to taste

Method:

Make sure your potatoes are all a similar size and cook in salted boiling water for 10 mins, or until just tender. Heat a little low cal spray in a frying pan and gently sauté the cumin seeds, mustard seeds, chilli flakes and onion for a few minutes. Add the shredded cabbages and cook for another 2-3 minutes. Season and add the cooked salad potatoes, coconut cream and lemon juice. Warm everything through and serve with chopped coriander sprinkled over the top.

Aromatic Spiced Cauliflower

Serves: 1 Calories: 181

Ingredients:

½ onion, sliced

½ tsp each ground ginger, cumin & tumeric

½ tsp garam masala

1 green chilli, sliced

1 garlic clove , crushed

¼ head large cauliflower

60ml/ ¼ cup vegetable stock/broth

1 tbsp fat-free natural yogurt

1 tsp ground almonds

Salt & pepper to taste

Method:

Add a little low cal cooking oil to a pan and gently sauté
the onions, green chilli and garlic. Mix the dry spices with
a teaspoon of water to make a paste and add to the
onions. Break the cauliflower into very small florets and
add to the onion spice mix in the pan. Add the stock,
cover and leave to simmer for 5-7 minutes, or until the
cauliflower is tender. Add the yoghurt and almonds,
season, stir and gently warm through for a few minutes.
Serve immediately.

Oyster Sauce Aubergine

Serves: 1 Calories: 140

Ingredients:

1 small aubergine, cut into 10 long wedges

2 spring onions/scallions, sliced into thin strips

1 red chillies, deseeded and sliced into strips

2 tsp black bean sauce

2 tsp oyster sauce

1 tsp lime juice

1 tbsp fresh chopped coriander/cilantro leaves

Low cal cooking spray

Salt & pepper to taste

Method:

Plunge the aubergine wedges into a pan of salted boiling water for 2 minutes. Drain and dry off.

Heat a little low cal spray in a frying pan and brown the aubergine wedges. Add the rest of the ingredients (except chopped coriander) and toss on the heat for 2-3 minutes. Sprinkle with coriander leaves and serve.

Fennel & Basil Linguine

Serves: 1 Calories: 195

Ingredients:

½ chopped fennel bulb & ½ tsp fennel seeds

½ onion, ½ carrot & ¼ red pepper, sliced

1 garlic clove, crushed

1 tbsp tomato purée/paste

100g/ 3½oz tinned chopped tomatoes

120ml/ ½ cup vegetable stock/broth

50g/2oz linguine pasta

pinch each sugar & crushed chilli flakes

1 tbsp fresh chopped basil

Low cal cooking spray

Salt & pepper to taste

Method:

Gently sauté the peppers, garlic, fennel, onion and carrot in a little low cal spray for 5-7 mins. Add the chilli flakes, fennel seeds, tomato purée, tomatoes, stock and sugar. Season and simmer for 10-15 mins until everything is well cooked. Meanwhile cook the linguine in salted boiling water until tender, drain and add to the frying pan. Simmer on a high heat for a few minutes to reduce the liquid. Sprinkle with chopped basil and serve.

Garlic Porcini 'Rice'

Serves: 1 Calories: 195

Ingredients:

½ onion, chopped

2 garlic cloves, crushed

1 tbsp balsamic vinegar

60ml/¼ cup vegetable stock/broth

3 tbsp dried porcini mushrooms, rehydrated and finely chopped

100g/3 ½oz mushrooms, sliced

½ cauliflower

Salt & Pepper to taste

1 tbsp chopped fresh flat leaf parsley

Low cal cooking spray

Salt & pepper to taste

Method:

In a food processor whizz the cauliflower until it is the size of rice grains. In a frying pan sauté the onion, garlic and mushrooms in a little low cal spray for a few minutes. Add the stock and vinegar then stir and season well. Cook for 3 minutes and add the cauliflower 'rice'. Cook until the liquid is reduced, the mushrooms cooked and the cauliflower tender. Serve sprinkled with flat leaf parsley.

Soups Under 200 Calories

Soups are a great, filling, wholesome meal choice. These recipes are all individual portions, but more often than not it makes sense to prepare larger batches of soup and save in single servings for another time. If you do decide you want make multiple servings just increase the quantities evenly across the ingredients.

Soups can also be 'filled' out by adding a little more stock or skimmed milk to give additional quantity with very little added calories.

Soups make a great warming lunch when you are at work and can easily be made in advance to heat up when you need it

Try having one of the lower calorie soups as a snack in a thermo-mug to sip on while you are travelling or watching TV

Tuscan Bean Soup

Serves: 1 Calories: 179

Ingredients:

½ onion, chopped

1 garlic clove, crushed

1 stick celery, chopped

1 courgette/zucchini, chopped

100g/3 ½ oz chopped tomatoes (tinned or fresh)

310ml/ 1 ¼ cups vegetable stock/broth

100g/ 3 ½ oz tinned mixed beans

½ tsp dried oregano

½ tsp dried basil

1 tbsp tomato puree/paste

1 tsp flat leaf parsley, chopped

Salt & pepper to taste

Method:

Place everything in a saucepan, except the parsley, beans & courgette. Simmer for 10 minutes. Add the chopped beans and courgettes and heat through for another 5 minutes or until all the vegetables and tender and cooked through. Season and serve with the chopped parsley sprinkled on top.

Red Pepper & Yoghurt Soup

Serves: 1 Calories: 111

Ingredients:

75g/3oz red peppers/bell peppers, chopped

½ onion, chopped

½ red chilli, deseeded and chopped

120ml/ ½ cup tomato passatta/sieved tomatoes

120ml/ ½ cup vegetable broth/stock

1 tsp dried basil

1 tsp chopped fresh dill

Salt & pepper to taste

60ml/ ¼ cup low fat yoghurt

Method:

Bring all the ingredients, except the chopped basil and yoghurt, to the boil in a saucepan. Cover and leave to simmer for 20 minutes. When the vegetables are tender use a blender or food processor to blend the soup into a smooth consistency. Adjust the seasoning and serve with the yoghurt gently dolloped into the centre of the bowl and the fresh dill sprinkled on top.

Beetroot Soup

Serves: 1 Calories: 149

Ingredients:

½ onion chopped

75g/3oz potato, chopped

½ small cooking apple, peeled, cored and chopped

1 tbsp water

½ tsp dried cumin

½ tsp dried coriander/cillantro

125g/4oz fresh cooked beetroot, diced

½ tsp lemon juice

250ml/1 cup veg stock/broth

1 tbsp low fat crème fraiche

Salt & pepper to taste

Method:

Add all the ingredients, except the crème fraiche and lemon, into a saucepan and bring to the boil. Cover and leave to simmer for 20 minutes. When the vegetables are tender use a blender, or food processor, to blend the soup into a smooth consistency. Stir through the lemon juice and adjust the seasoning. Serve with the crème fraiche gently swirled through.

Spicy Apricot & Apple Soup

Serves: 1 Calories: 182

Ingredients:

40g/ 1 ½ oz dried apricots, (soaked in water over night and chopped)

125g/4 oz apples, cored, peeled & chopped

½ onion, chopped

1 tsp lime juice

250ml/1 cup vegetable stock/broth

Pinch of nutmeg & cinnamon

½ tsp dried cumin

¼ tsp chilli powder (optional)

1 tbsp low fat yoghurt

Salt & Pepper to taste

Method:

Add all the ingredients, except the yoghurt and lime juice, into a saucepan and bring to the boil. Cover and leave to simmer for 20 minutes. When the vegetables are tender, use a blender or food processor to blend the soup into a smooth consistency. Stir through the lime juice and adjust the seasoning. Serve with the yoghurt dolloped on top.

Spiced Pea Soup

Serves: 1 Calories: 198

Ingredients:

½ onion, chopped

50g/2oz potatoes, peeled & chopped

1 clove garlic, crushed

½ tsp each ground coriander/cilantro, cumin & ginger

250ml/1 cup vegetable stock/broth

125g/4oz frozen peas

1 tsp chopped fresh mint

60ml/ ¼ cup skimmed milk

1 tbsp low fat yoghurt

Low cal cooking spray

Method:

Gently sauté the onions and potato in a little low cal spray until the onion begins to soften. Add the garlic and dried spices and stir for a minute or two. Add the stock and peas, cover and leave to simmer for 15 minutes or until the potatoes are tender. Use a blender or food processor to blend the soup into a smooth consistency. Return to the pan and add the milk. Warm through, take off the heat, add the yoghurt and stir through. Adjust the seasoning and sprinkle with the chopped mint.

Mushroom & Noodle Soup

Serves: 1 Calories: 166

Ingredients:

50g/2oz fresh mushrooms, sliced

250ml/1 cup vegetable stock/broth

75g/3oz fine egg noodles

1 garlic clove, crushed

½ tsp ground ginger

1 tsp soy sauce

75g/3oz beansprouts

½ onion, chopped

1 tsp each ketchup & fresh chopped coriander/cilantro,

Salt & pepper to taste

Low cal cooking spray

Method:

Gently sauté the mushrooms, garlic and onion in a little low cal spray. When the onion softens add the ginger and stir through, cooking for a minute or two longer. Place in a pan with the stock, noodles, soy sauce and ketchup. Season, cover and simmer for 5-10 minutes until the noodles are tender. Add the beansprouts and warm for a minute or two. Adjust the seasoning and serve with the chopped coriander sprinkled over the top.

Carrot & Fresh Coriander Soup

Serves: 1 Calories: 125

Ingredients:

½ onion, chopped

½ tsp ground coriander/cilantro

75g/3oz potatoes, peeled & chopped

125g/4oz carrots, peeled & chopped

250ml/1 cup vegetable/broth

3 tbsp fresh chopped coriander/cilantro

Low cal cooking oil

Salt & pepper to taste

Method:

Heat a little low cal spray in a frying pan and gently sauté the onion for a few minutes. Add the ground coriander, potato, carrots and stock. Season, cover and leave to simmer for 20 mins or until the carrots are tender. Pulse the soup in a food processor until smooth. Stir through the chopped coriander and serve.

Chickpea & Cumin Soup

Serves: 1 Calories: 166

Ingredients:

½ onion, chopped

½ clove garlic, crushed

1 stick celery, chopped

1 tsp ground cumin

150ml/1 cup vegetable stock/broth

125g/4oz chopped tomatoes with garlic

125g/4oz tinned chickpeas

1 tsp lemon juice

1 tbsp chopped flat leaf parsley

Low cal cooking oil

Salt & pepper to taste

Method:

Heat a little low cal spray in a frying pan and gently sauté the onion and celery for a few minutes. Add the cumin, stock, tomatoes and chickpeas. Cover and leave to simmer for 10 minutes or until everything is tender. Season, stir through lemon juice, sprinkle with parsley and serve.

Thai Lemongrass & Squash Soup

Serves: 1 Calories: 191

Ingredients:

250g/9oz Butternut Squash flesh, cubed

½ onion, chopped

¼ tsp ground ginger

1 lemongrass stalk, bashed

2 tsp each Thai red curry paste & lime juice

60ml/ ¼ cup low fat coconut milk

250ml/1 cup vegetable stock/broth

½ red chilli, finely sliced

Low cal cooking oil

Salt & pepper to taste

Method:

Pre heat oven to 200C/180C fan/gas 6. Spray the squash with a little low cal cooking oil and roast for 20mins or until tender. Meanwhile sauté the onion, chilli, ginger and lemongrass in a little low cal spray for a few minutes. Add the curry paste, stock and roasted squash. Cover, season and leave to simmer for a few minutes. Remove the lemongrass and pulse the soup in a food processor until smooth. Add the lime juice and coconut milk, gently heat through and serve.

Spinach & Cream Soup

Serves: 1 Calories: 186

Ingredients

2 spring onions/scallions, chopped

½ leek, sliced

1 stick celery, sliced

50g/2oz small potato, peeled and diced

½ tsp ground black pepper

250ml/1 cup vegetable stock/broth

150g/5oz spinach

60ml/ ¼ cup single cream

Low cal cooking oil

Salt & pepper to taste

Method:

Gently sauté the spring onions, leek, celery and potato in a little low cal spray. Add the stock, cover and leave to simmer for 7-8 minutes until the potatoes are tender. Add the spinach, cook for 2 minutes and pulse in a food processor until smooth. Season, stir in the cream, gently heat and serve.

THE Skinny
5:2 FAST DIET
MEALS FOR one

VEGETARIAN

Smoothies Under 200 Calories

Smoothies are a fantastic way to supplement your 5:2 Diet fast days. A smoothie is basically a thick blended drink which in addition to fruit or vegetables usually includes crushed ice, yoghurt or milk (or milk alternative). Smoothies can be a fantastic source of vitamins and nutrients and they taste great. They help make up the essential daily intake of fruit (and veg) and unlike many of the store bought drinks, the following recipes contain no added sugar and all fall under 100 or 200 calories.

Tips For A Perfect Smoothie

Everyone has their own tips for how to make the perfect smoothie and indeed you should experiment and take advice from lots of different sources to find what works best for you. To start you off follow our top tips for whizzing up the best smoothies first time around.

Add your liquid first, not fruit, to prevent your blender blade becoming blunt or damaged.

Freeze your fruit. If you want to save time in preparation you can freeze your favourite fruits in advance. Pretty much all fruit is fine to freeze for smoothies. Plus you won't need to use as much ice when you blend.

Choose good quality, seasonal and if possible organic fruit. Seasonal fruit will have a much stronger flavour and organic fruit should be free from any chemicals or preservatives. Freezing keeps all the goodness locked inside.

Avoid adding too many sweeteners such as sugar, ice cream etc. Most fruits have natural sweetness in them. Use natural sweetener such as Agave syrup, honey or Maple syrup if you can.

Blender Advice

A blender is an essential piece of kit for making smoothies. Some use a blending attachment to their mixer or others a stand-alone appliance – both will do the job.

How smooth do you like your smoothie? If you prefer a super smooth consistency then perhaps a blender with more power may be better for you.

Speed – do you need multiple speeds on your blender? For most, one setting will do the job nicely but as before if you prefer a smoother consistency you may wish to consider multiple speed settings.

Cleaning - Your blender will need a good clean after each use. You will generally need to remove the blade to do this – some blenders are simpler to reassemble than others. If you use a dishwasher makes sure the blender parts are dishwasher safe. Another good tip is to use freshly squeezed lemon juice all over to help zap those stubborn marks.

Breakfast Smoothie

Serves: 1 Calories: 120

Ingredients:
140g/4 ½ oz blackberries
120ml/ ½ cup apple juice
½ banana
Handful of ice cubes

Method:
Combine all the ingredients into a blender and blend until smooth.

Raspberry & Almond Milk Smoothie

Serves: 1 Calories: 116

Ingredients:
120ml/ ½ cup almond milk
100g/3 ½ oz raspberries
½ banana

½ tbsp agave nectar
Handful of ice cubes

Method:
Combine all the ingredients into a blender and blend until smooth.

Cherry Hit Smoothie

Serves: 1 Calories: 193

Ingredients:
125g/4oz cherries
1 kiwi fruit
60 ml/ ¼ cup pure orange juice
60 ml/ ¼ cup coconut water
½ tbsp agave nectar
Handful of ice

Method:
Combine all the ingredients into a blender and blend until smooth.

Peach, Apple & Cucumber Smoothie

Serves: 1 Calories: 143

Ingredients:
1 medium peach, peeled and stoned
60ml/ ¼ cup pure apple juice
20g/3/4oz cucumber, peeled
2 tsp lime juice
1 tsp fresh mint, finely chopped
1 tbsp agave nectar
2 handfuls of ice

Method:
Combine all the ingredients into a blender and blend until smooth.

Tropical Smoothie

Serves: 1 Calories: 169

Ingredients:
1 mango, peeled and stoned
½ banana
60ml/ ½ cup fat free peach yoghurt
60ml/ ½ cup cranberry juice
Handful Of ice

Method:
Combine all the ingredients into a blender and blend until smooth.

Blueberry Banana Smoothie

Serves: 1 Calories: 195

Ingredients:
150g/5oz blueberries
1 banana
120ml/ ½ cup pineapple juice
Handful of ice

Method:
Combine all the ingredients into a blender and blend until smooth.

Ginger & Strawberry Smoothie

Serves: 1 Calories: 195

Ingredients:
120ml/ ½ cup skimmed milk
1 banana
75g/3oz strawberries
1 tsp fresh ginger finely chopped
1 tsp agave nectar
Handful of ice

Method:
Combine all the ingredients into a blender and blend until smooth.

Pomegranate, Kiwi & Berry Smoothie

Serves: 1 Calories: 189

Ingredients:
½ banana
1 kiwi, peeled
75g/3oz blueberries
75g/3oz strawberries
120ml/ ½ cup cranberry juice
Handful of ice

Method:
Combine all the ingredients into a blender and blend until smooth.

Peach & Ginger Smoothie

Serves: 1 Calories: 160

Ingredients:
2 medium peaches, skinned and stoned
120ml/ ½ cup unsweetened apple juice
½ tsp ground ginger
1 tsp agave nectar
Handful of ice

Method:
Combine all the ingredients into a blender and blend until smooth.

Strawberry Spinach Smoothie

Serves: 1
Calories: 157

Ingredients:
1 banana

100g/3 ½ oz strawberries
25g/1oz fresh spinach leaves
60ml/ ¼ cup fat free vanilla yoghurt
1 tsp honey
Handful of ice

Method:
Combine all the ingredients into a blender and blend until smooth.

Cranberry & Apple Smoothie

Serves: 1 Calories: 150

Ingredients:
75g/3oz blueberries
75g/3oz strawberries
1 small apple, cored and chopped
75g/3oz fresh cranberries
1 tsp honey
Handful of ice

Method:
Combine all the ingredients into a blender and blend until smooth.

Spiced Up Banana Smoothie

Serves: 1 Calories: 144

Ingredients:
1 banana
120ml/ ½ cup skimmed milk
¼ tsp ground cinnamon
¼ tsp ground nutmeg
¼ tsp ground cloves
Handful of ice

Method:
Combine all the ingredients into a blender and blend until smooth.

Rhubarb Smoothie

Serves: 1 Calories: 188

Ingredients:
2 rhubarb stalks, trimmed and chopped
60ml/ ¼ cup orange juice
60ml/ ¼ cup fat free plain yoghurt
1 tbsp agave nectar
Handful of ice

Method:
Combine all the ingredients into a blender and blend until smooth.

Green Veg Smoothie

Serves: 1 Calories: 88

Ingredients:
60g/2 ½ oz broccoli
40g/1 ½ oz cucumber
120ml/ ½ cup fat free yoghurt
1 tbsp lime juice
4 tbsp pineapple juice
Handful of ice

Method:
Bring a pan of water to the boil and add the broccoli florets. Cook for 5-6 mins or until tender.
Remove from the heat, drain and cool. Place the yoghurt, broccoli, cucumber, lime, pineapple juice and ice into blender and blend until smooth.

Spinach, Grape & Kiwi Smoothie

Serves: 1 Calories: 100

Ingredients:
75g/3oz green grapes
1 kiwi, peeled

25g/1oz spinach, stalk removed
120ml/ ½ cup watermelon juice
Handful of ice

Method:
Combine all the ingredients into a blender and blend until smooth.

Vanilla & Banana Smoothie

Serves: 1 Calories: 95

Ingredients:
½ banana
120ml/ ½ cup fat free vanilla yoghurt
Handful of ice

Method:
Combine all the ingredients into a blender and blend until smooth.

Coffee Smoothie

Serves: 1 Calories: 168

Ingredients:
60ml/ ¼ cup black brewed coffee
1 banana
120ml/ ½ cup fat free plain yoghurt
75g/3oz strawberries
¼ tsp cinnamon
½ tbsp cocoa powder

Method:
Combine all the ingredients into a blender and blend until smooth.

Strawberry & Banana Smoothie

Serves: 1 Calories: 120

Ingredients:

120ml/ ½ cup plain fat free yoghurt
½ banana
5 strawberries
Handful of ice

Method:
Combine all the ingredients into a blender and blend until smooth.

Mixed Berry Smoothie

Serves: 1 Calories: 130

Ingredients:
½ banana
200g/7oz mixed berries
120ml/ ½ cup plain fat free yoghurt
Handful of ice.

Method:
Combine all the ingredients into a blender and blend until smooth.

Kiwi & Strawberry Smoothie

Serves: 1 Calories: 120

Ingredients:
1 banana
1 kiwi fruit
5 strawberries
1 tsp agave nectar
60ml/1/2 cup skimmed milk
Handful of ice

Method:
Combine all the ingredients into a blender and blend until smooth.

THE
Skinny
5:2 FAST DIET
MEALS FOR
one

VEGETARIAN

Recipes Under 300 Calories

Healthy Club Sandwich

Serves: 1 Calories: 270

Ingredients:

2 slices granary bread

50g/2oz rocket

1 carrot

1 tsp lemon juice

2 tbsp low fat houmous

2 tomatoes, chopped

Salt & pepper to taste

Method:

Lightly toast the granary bread and spread the houmous over both slices. Grate the carrot and place in a bowl with the lemon juice, rocket and chopped tomatoes. Season well and load onto one of the houmous covered granary slices. Top with the other slice, cut in half and serve.

Veggie Chickpea & Pumpkin Curry

Serves: 1 Calories: 281

Ingredients:

2 tsp Thai yellow curry paste

250g/7oz pumpkin flesh, cubed

120ml/½ cup each veg stock/broth & low fat coconut milk

75g/3oz tinned chickpeas

½ onion, sliced

1 stalk lemongrass

1 tsp mustard seed

1 tbsp lime juice

1 tbsp fresh chopped coriander/cilantro

Salt & pepper to taste

Low cal cooking spray

Method:

Gently sauté the onion and mustard seeds in a little low cal spray. Take the tip off the lemongrass stalk and bash with a rolling pin to release the flavour. Add the curry paste and lemongrass; cook for a few minutes. Add the pumpkin, chickpeas and stock; cover and leave to simmer for 8-10 minutes, or until the pumpkin is tender. Add the coconut milk and gently warm through. Serve with chopped coriander/cilantro sprinkled over the top.

Sun Blush Barley Salad

Serves: 1 Calories: 299

Ingredients:

200g/7oz butternut squash flesh, cubed

40g/1½ oz pearl barley & 5 chopped black olives

100g/3½ oz purple sprouting broccoli, roughly chopped

25g/1oz sun blush tomatoes, finely sliced

1 tsp capers & ½ crushed garlic clove

50g/2oz watercress & 1 tbsp chopped fresh basil

1 tbsp balsamic vinegar & 1 tsp olive oil & Dijon mustard

Salt & pepper to taste

Low cal cooking spray

Method:

Pre-heat the oven to 200C/fan 180C/gas 6.

Place the barley in a pan of salted boiling water and leave to cook for 20 mins or until the barley is tender. Drain and leave to cool. Spray the squash with low cal cooking oil and roast for 20 mins or until tender. Combine together the olive oil, balsamic vinegar, Dijon mustard and garlic. Cook the broccoli for 2 mins in boiling water. Drain and combine with the barley, tomatoes, squash, olive oil dressing, olives, capers & watercress. Serve with chopped basil sprinkled over the top.

Sugar Snap & Soya Bean Salad

Serves: 1 Calories: 291

Ingredients:

40g/1 ½ oz puy lentils

Pinch crushed chilli flakes

1 tsp each sesame oil & ground ginger

1 tbsp lemon juice & 2 tbsp soy sauce

½ garlic clove, crushed & 1 tsp runny honey

250ml/1 cup vegetable stock/broth

75g/3oz young tender stem broccoli, roughly chopped

40g/1½ oz each fresh soya beans & sugar snap peas

1 tbsp fresh chopped oregano

Salt & pepper to taste

Method:

Make sure the stock is boiling hot and add the puy lentils. Cook for 15 mins or until tender, then drain. Meanwhile, add the broccoli, soya beans and sugar snap peas to a pan of boiling salted water and cook for 2-3 minutes until al dente. Drain and add to the cooling puy lentils. Combine the sesame oil, honey, chilli flakes, lemon juice, garlic, ginger and soy sauce. Tip onto the lentil mix and combine gently to coat everything with the dressing. Season and serve with the chopped oregano over the top.

Fresh Herb Pitta

Serves: 1 Calories: 292

Ingredients:

150g/5oz frozen broad beans

½ cucumber

2 mini (10g/ ½ oz) wholemeal pitta breads

1 tbsp lemon juice

1 tsp olive oil

Pinch caster sugar

1 tbsp fresh chopped mint

1 tbsp fresh chopped flat leaf parsley

1 tbsp fresh chopped chives

Method:

Combine together the lemon juice, olive oil, sugar and seasoning.

Chop the cucumber into small cubes. Cook the broad beans in a pan of salted boiling water for approx. 3 minutes or until tender; drain and leave to cool. Add the chopped cucumber to the beans in a shallow bowl and combine with the dressing. Cut the mini pitta breads into diagonal strips and arrange in the bowl with the beans. Serve sprinkled with the mint, parsley & chives.

Halloumi Watermelon Salad

Serves: 1 Calories: 277

Ingredients:

50g/2oz halloumi cheese, thinly sliced

250g/9oz watermelon flesh, cubed

50g/2oz fresh peas

75g/3oz baby courgettes/zucchini

1 tbsp lemon juice

1 tsp olive oil

1 tbsp chopped fresh mint

½ tsp crushed chilli flakes

Method:

Preheat the grill to medium/high.

Slice the baby courgettes lengthways and place on the grill, flesh side up, beside the sliced halloumi cheese. Season both well, sprinkle with chilli flakes and spray with a little low cal cooking spray.

Grill for 2-3 minutes each side or until golden. In a bowl mix together the mint, olive oil, cubed watermelon, fresh peas (eat these raw) and lemon juice. Arrange on a plate with the cheese and courgettes/zucchini.

Spicy Coconut Potatoes

Serves: 1 Calories: 246

Ingredients:

½ onion, chopped

75g/3oz potatoes, peeled and cubed

½ aubergine/egg plant, cubed

120g/4oz mushrooms, sliced

2 tsp curry powder

½ tsp paprika

60ml/¼ cup vegetable stock

120ml/ ½ cup low fat coconut milk

1 tbsp fresh chopped coriander/cilantro

Low cal cooking spray

Method:

Gently sauté the onion in a little low cal cooking spray for a few minutes. Add the curry powder and paprika to a little water to make a paste and add this to the onions cooking in the pan. Add the potatoes and stock; cover and leave to simmer for a few minutes. Add the mushrooms and aubergine and cook for a further few minutes until everything is tender. Add the coconut milk and warm through. Serve with the chopped coriander sprinkled on top.

Moroccan Spinach Chickpeas

Serves: 1 Calories: 270

Ingredients:

1 onion, chopped

125g/4oz courgettes/zucchini, sliced

¼ tsp each ground cinnamon, turmeric, coriander/cilantro and cumin

1 fresh tomato, chopped

100g/3½oz each tinned chickpeas & fresh spinach

1 tbsp raisins

120ml/½ cup vegetable stock/broth

75g/3oz frozen peas

1 tbsp fresh chopped mint

Salt & pepper to taste

Low cal cooking spray

Method:

Gently sauté the onion and courgettes in a little low cal spray for a few minutes. Stir in the dried spices and chopped tomato. Season and add the chickpeas, raisins, peas and stock. Cover and leave to simmer for 5-10 minutes or until everything is tender and warmed through. Stir in the spinach and cook for a further minute. Sprinkle with fresh mint and serve.

Pea & Mint Risotto

Serves: 1 Calories: 277

Ingredients:

½ onion, chopped

100g/3 ½oz frozen peas

500ml/2 cups vegetable stock/broth

75g/3oz risotto rice

1 tsp grated parmesan cheese

1 tbsp chopped fresh mint

Salt & pepper to taste

Low cal cooking spray

Method:

Gently sauté the onion in a little low cal cooking spray for a few minutes. Add the risotto rice and stir well. Add about a quarter of the stock to the rice, stirring and allowing the rice to absorb before adding more. Add the peas and chopped mint; keep on going for about 15 minutes until the risotto is tender. Season, sprinkle with parmesan and serve.

Pasta Salad

Serves: 1 Calories: 289

Ingredients:

75g/3 oz fusilli pasta

50g/2oz frozen peas

5 chopped black olives, finely chopped (optional)

2 chopped sundried tomatoes, finely chopped (optional)

1 tbsp balsamic vinegar

1 tbsp fresh chopped flat leaf parsley

1 tbsp lemon juice

2 tsp low fat mayo

Method:

Cook the fusilli in boiling salted water until tender, add the peas to the pan 5 minutes before the end of cooking time. Drain and leave to cool. Mix together the black olives, tomatoes, vinegar, mayonnaise and lemon juice to make a creamy dressing. Season and combine with the cooling pasta and peas. Serve with chopped parsley sprinkled over the top.

Egg & Mushroom Hash

Serves: 1 Calories: 286

Ingredients:

125g/4oz potatoes, diced

½ onion, chopped

½ tsp crushed chilli flakes

1 tsp olive oil

1 tsp dried basil or rosemary

50g/2oz mushrooms, chopped

1 medium free range egg

Method:

Pre-heat the oven to 200C/fan 180C/gas 6. Mix the chopped onion, potato and mushrooms in a bowl with the olive oil, seasoning, chilli flakes and dried herbs. Spread out into a small shallow ovenproof dish and cook for 15-20 minutes or until the potatoes are tender. Make a well in the middle of the potatoes and crack the egg in. Return to the oven and cook for another few minutes until the egg is cooked as you like it. Eat straight out of the oven dish.

Wholemeal, Cottage-Cheese & Peppers

Serves: 1 Calories: 240

Ingredients:

150g/5oz low fat cottage cheese

½ red pepper, sliced

1 tsp chopped fresh basil leaves

1 slice wholemeal bread

1 tsp balsamic vinegar

Low cal cooking spray

Method:

Gently sauté the peppers in a little low cal cooking spray. Season and add the balsamic vinegar. Increase the heat so that the vinegar reduces and the peppers become sticky. Toast the bread and plate up with the cottage cheese on top. Tip the peppers and balsamic juice on the top, sprinkle with basil and serve.

Tofu Hash

Serves: 1 Calories: 294

Ingredients:

½ red onion, sliced

½ carrot, peeled and diced

15g/ ½oz green beans

50g/2oz potatoes, peeled and diced

120ml/½ cup vegetable stock/broth

50g/2oz tofu, diced

1 tsp plain/general flour

1 tbsp fresh chopped flat leaf parsley

Salt & Pepper to taste

Low cal cooking oil

Method:

Sauté the onion, carrots, green beans and potatoes in a little low cal spray for a few minutes. Stir the flour into the vegetables and cook for another minute or two. Add the stock and simmer for 10 minutes or until the potatoes are tender. Add the tofu and gently heat through until all the stock has been absorbed. Season and serve with chopped parsley.

Spicy Potato Salad

Serves: 1 Calories: 241

Ingredients:

100g/3 ½oz salad potatoes

¼ avocado

2 tsp lemon juice

½ garlic clove, crushed

1 beefsteak/heirloom tomato, sliced

½ red chilli, chopped

1 yellow pepper/bell pepper, sliced

4 spring onions/scallions

½ tsp olive oil

1 tbsp fresh chopped coriander/cilantro

Salt & Pepper to taste

Method:

Cook the salad potatoes in salted boing water for 8-10 minutes or until tender. Put to one side to cool. Meanwhile mash the avocado flesh with the chopped chillies, lemon juice, garlic and seasoning. Place the potatoes, sliced tomatoes, peppers, spring onions and olive oil in a bowl. Toss well and season. Arrange on a plate and then load the avocado mixture on top. Sprinkle with chopped coriander and serve.

Rice Salad

Serves: 1 Calories: 294

Ingredients:

½ onion & ½ red chilli, finely chopped

½ tsp each turmeric, cumin & garam masala

75g/3oz each long grain rice & cauliflower

1 large tomato, chopped

25g/1oz raisins

1 cup vegetable stock/broth

½ red pepper/bell pepper, sliced

1 tsp grated almonds

Salt & pepper to taste

Low cal cooking oil

Method:

Break the cauliflower into small florets. Gently sauté with the onion, cumin, turmeric, garam masala, chopped tomatoes and sliced peppers in a little low cal spray for a few minutes. Add the rice to the pan, stir and pour the stock into the pan. Cover and leave to simmer for 15-20 minutes or until the rice is tender and the stock absorbed (add a little water during cooking if needed). Add the raisins, warm through, season and serve with grated almonds sprinkled over the top.

Aloo Gobi

Serves: 1 Calories: 250

Ingredients:

½ cauliflower, split into florets

200g/7oz tinned chopped tomatoes

½ onion, chopped

Handful of shredded green cabbage

100g/3½oz peeled diced potatoes

1 tbsp fresh chopped coriander/cilantro

½ tsp each chilli powder, garlic powder, ground ginger, sugar, garam masala & ground cumin

1 tsp turmeric

½ tsp salt

Low cal cooking spray

Method:

Add a little low cal spray to a frying pan and gently sauté the onions. Mix in the dried spices, salt and fresh coriander and cook for a further minute or two. Next add the sugar, cabbage, chopped tomatoes, cauliflower and potatoes, cover and cook on the lowest possible setting for at about 20 minutes. Make sure the vegetables are completely tender before serving.

Mixed Vegetable Curry

Serves: 1 Calories: 207

Ingredients:

100g/3½oz frozen peas

½ carrot, peeled & cut into batons

½ onion, chopped

50g/2oz spinach, chopped

¼ cauliflower, broken into florets

50g/2oz potato cubed

100g/3 ½ oz chopped tomatoes

1 tbsp tomato puree/paste

½ tsp cumin, turmeric & coriander

1 tsp mild curry powder

½ tsp each mild chilli powder & salt

Low cal cooking spray

Method:

Heat a little low cal spray in a frying pan and gently sauté the onion. After a few minutes add the other vegetables and continue to cook. Mix the dry spices in a little water and add to the pan along with the salt and chopped tomatoes. Cover and leave to cook gently until all the vegetables are tender.

Spiced Okra & 'Rice'

Serves: 1 Calories: 231

Ingredients:

1 tsp olive oil

2 onions, sliced

125g/4oz okra, trimmed and sliced

100g/3 ½ oz tinned chopped tomatoes

½ tsp chilli powder

½ tsp tumeric

1 tsp ground coriander/cilantro

1 tbsp fresh chopped coriander/cilantro

¼ large head cauliflower

Salt & Pepper to taste

Method:

Whizz the cauliflower in a food processor until it is the size of rice grains.

Heat the oil in a frying pan and gently sauté the onions, okra, chilli powder, turmeric, tomatoes and ground coriander. Cook for 5 minutes, season and add the cauliflower 'rice'. Cook for a further 5 minutes until the 'rice' and vegetables are tender. Sprinkle with chopped coriander and serve.

Wild Mushroom & Garlic Penne

Serves: 1 Calories: 235

Ingredients:

125g/4oz wild mushrooms, sliced

1 tsp wholegrain mustard

2 garlic cloves, crushed

75g/3oz penne pasta

1 tbsp fresh chopped flat leaf parsley

1 tsp lemon juice

1 tbsp low-fat cream cheese

60ml/ ¼ cup vegetable stock/broth

Salt & pepper to taste

Method:

Pour the stock, mushrooms, mustard and garlic into a frying pan and simmer for 5 minutes, or until the stock has reduced right down. Meanwhile cook the penne in boiling salted water until tender. Stir the cream cheese through the mushrooms. Add the pasta to the pan and combine well. Season, stir through the lemon juice and sprinkle with parsley to serve.

Tomato & Avocado Salad

Serves: 1 Calories: 230

Ingredients:

4 large vine ripened tomatoes, diced

Pinch of paprika

½ ripe avocado, diced

1 tsp red wine vinegar

1 tbsp balsamic vinegar

1 tbsp fresh chopped chives

½ red onion sliced

1 baby gem lettuce, shredded

Salt & pepper to taste

Method:

Mix together the vinegars and pour over the diced avocado, lettuce, tomato and onion; toss well. Sprinkle the paprika and chives on top.

Courgette & Pea Couscous

Serves: 1 Calories: 210

Ingredients:

100g/3 ½ oz couscous

50g/2oz frozen peas

50g/2oz courgette/zuchinni, cubed

1 tsp dried basil

120ml/ ½ cup vegetable stock/broth

1 tomato, chopped

1 tbsp lemon juice

Low cal spray

Salt & pepper to taste

Method:

Place the couscous, dried basil and frozen peas into a bowl and pour the stock in; leave covered.

Meanwhile sauté the courgette in a little low cal spray for a few minutes. Remove from the heat and mix with the tomatoes and lemon juice; season well. After 4-6 minutes, check the couscous is tender and the peas cooked through. Drain any excess liquid and fluff with a fork. Toss in a bowl with the courgette and tomatoes.

Sticky Peanut Noodles

Serves: 1 Calories: 288

Ingredients:

1 tbsp chopped peanuts

70g/3oz straight-to-wok egg noodles

1 tsp runny honey

2 tsp lemon juice

1 tbsp soy sauce

120ml/ ½ cup vegetable stock/broth

50g/2oz courgette/zucchini, peeled into ribbons

½ carrot & ½ red pepper cut into matchsticks

Pinch of sesame seeds

Low cal cooking spray

Salt & pepper to taste

Method:

Saute the courgette ribbons in a frying pan with a little low cal cooking spray for a few minutes. Mix together the honey, lemon, stock and soy in a cup. Add the carrots and peppers to the courgette pan and fry for a minute longer. Add the liquid in the cup to the pan, along with the noodles and cook for 5 minutes or until the vegetables are tender and the noodles warmed through. Sprinkle with the peanuts and sesame seeds then serve straight away.

Fresh Pea Linguine

Serves: 1 Calories: 271

Ingredients:

75g/3oz linguine pasta

75g/3oz fresh sugar snap peas

25g/1oz rocket

1 garlic clove, crushed

½ red chilli, deseeded and finely chopped

4 cherry tomatoes, halved

1 tbsp fresh chopped basil

1 tsp lime juice

½ tsp caster sugar

Salt & pepper to taste

Low cal cooking spray

Method:

Cook the linguine in boiling salted water until tender. Add the sugar snap peas to the pan 2 minutes before the end of cooking time. Drain and put to one side.

Meanwhile, gently sauté the tomatoes, chilli and garlic in a little low cal cooking spray; season and stir through the lime juice and sugar. Toss in the pasta and sugar snap peas. Sprinkle with chopped basil and serve.

Pak Choi Noodle Broth

Serves: 1 Calories: 214

Ingredients:

250ml/1 cup vegetable stock/broth

1 whole pak choi, shredded

75g/3oz straight to wok noodles

4 spring onions/scallions

2 tsp oyster sauce

2 tsp hoisin sauce

2 tsp soy sauce

1 tsp lime juice

½ tsp ground ginger

Method:

Add all the ingredients, except the spring onions, to a wok. Gently simmer for 4-5 minutes. Cut the spring onions lengthways into matchsticks. Tip the noodles into a bowl. Season and garnish with spring onion.

Scrambled Eggs & Watercress

Serves: 1 Calories: 225

Ingredients:

3 free range eggs

50g/2oz watercress

1 lemon wedge

2 crackerbread

1 tsp low fat olive spread

Pinch crushed chilli flakes

Salt & pepper to taste

Method:

Crack the eggs into a cup, lightly whisk and season well. Use ½ tsp olive spread to 'butter' the crackerbread. Heat the other ½ tsp olive spread in a small frying pan and tip in the eggs. Keep on stirring continuously on a med/high heat until the eggs are nearly cooked but still 'sloppy'. Add the watercress; quickly stir through and serve with black pepper, crackerbread and a pinch of chilli flakes.

Other CookNation Titles

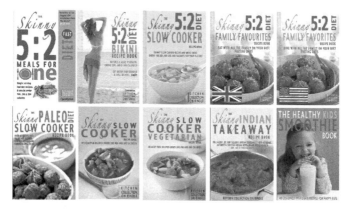

You may also be interested in other titles in the CookNation series:

The Skinny 5:2 Fast Diet Meals For One
Single Serving Fast Day Recipes & Snacks Under 100, 200 & 300 Calories

The Skinny 5:2 Bikini Diet Recipe Book
Recipes & Meal Planners Under 100, 200 & 300 Calories. Get Ready For Summer & Lose Weight... FAST!

The Skinny 5:2 Slow Cooker Recipe Book
Skinny Slow Cooker Recipe And Menu Ideas Under 100, 200, 300 & 400 Calories For Your 5:2 Diet.

The Skinny 5:2 Family Favourites Recipe Book
(UK & US Editions)
Eat With All the Family On Your Diet Fasting Days.

The Skinny Slow Cooker Recipe Book
40 Delicious Recipes Under 300, 400 And 500 Calories.

The Skinny Slow Cooker Vegetarian Recipe Book
40 Delicious Recipes Under 200, 300 And 400 Calories.

The Skinny Paleo Diet Slow Cooker Recipe Book
Over 40 Gluten Free Paleo Diet Recipes For Weight Loss
And Enhanced Well Being.

The Skinny Indian Takeaway Recipe Book
Authentic British Indian Restaurant Dishes Under 300, 400
And 500 Calories.

The Healthy Kids Smoothie Book
40 Delicious Goodness In A Glass Recipes for Happy
Kids.

Find all these great titles by searching under
'CookNation' on Amazon.

If you enjoyed The Skinny 5:2 Fast Diet Meals For One
we'd really appreciate your feedback. Reviews help others
decide if this is the right book for them so a moment of
your time would be appreciated. Thank you.